Take Charge of Your Eating

Take Charge of Your Eating

written by
Laura Pirott

illustrated by
R.W. Alley

ONE
CARING
PLACE

Abbey Press

Text © 2004 by Laura Pirott
Illustrations © 2004 by St. Meinrad Archabbey
Published by One Caring Place
Abbey Press
St. Meinrad, Indiana 47577

Library of Congress Catalog Number
2003113874

ISBN 978-0-87029-378-8

Printed in the United States of America

Foreword

Food keeps us physically alive, while also serving other important functions, both culturally and societally.

On the other hand, many of us turn to food when we feel confused, anxious, or hurt. At these times especially, we may care neither about the quantity nor the quality of the food. That's when we may hurt ourselves without consciously thinking about it, or live with the guilt and shame of our actions.

This refreshing and helpful book offers a view of food and eating that is quite different from the cultural standard—food is neither good nor bad, but neutral.

The book offers important tips on transforming negative energies and beliefs into positive benefits, promoting better habits and a healthier lifestyle. It uses a methodical and easy cleansing process that will support not only an improvement in health, but emotional and spiritual growth, as well.

1.

Look at your body and appreciate your physical uniqueness. Relax and be as you are, without trying to hide or wish away parts of yourself. God has lovingly made you. Marvel at the creation you are!

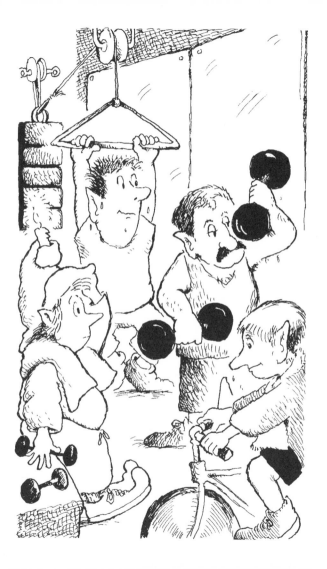

2.

Resist being seduced by fad diets and exercise programs that make extreme promises. Everyone is different. There is no "one-size-fits-all" technique. Listen to your body, your inner wisdom, for clues about what you may need to become healthier.

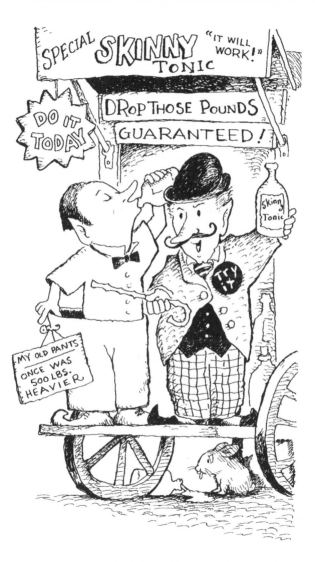

3.

Notice your own physical rhythms. How do you feel after you eat? Energized? Sluggish? Content? Do you burn food quickly, slowly, or in-between? What do you feel when you have dairy products, vegetables, meat, beans, fruit, grains, or processed foods? Only you have the answers to these questions.

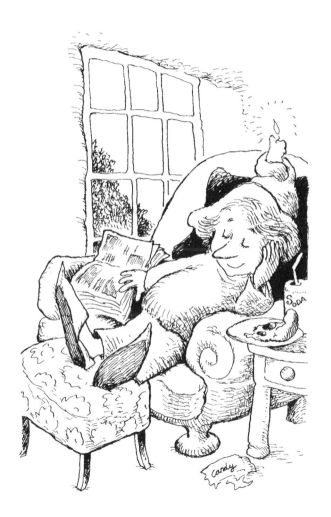

4.

Take charge of your eating habits. Educate yourself: read and talk to experts—inform yourself about nutrition and healthy living. Always consult your doctor before undertaking any major changes in your diet and/or exercise program.

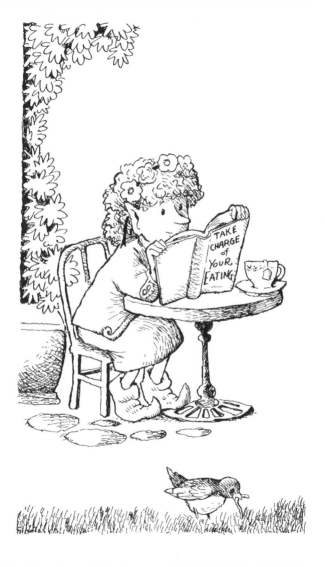

5.

Stay active! God designed our bodies to dance, run, play, jump, and stretch. Allow your body's energy to blossom by engaging in yoga, stretching, martial arts, sports, dance, and cardiovascular activity. Think of what you'd like to do and have fun!

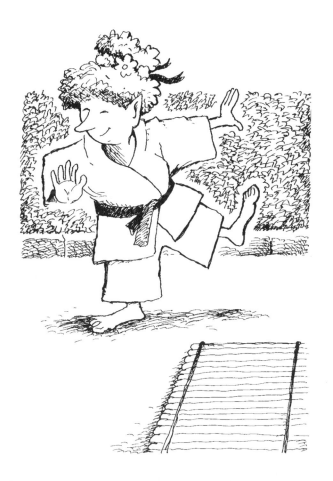

6.

Your heritage has a wealth of wisdom about food and nutrition. Learn from your family and participate in its traditions of food preparation. Share "secret" recipes from home with your co-workers and friends, and tell them some of your family stories.

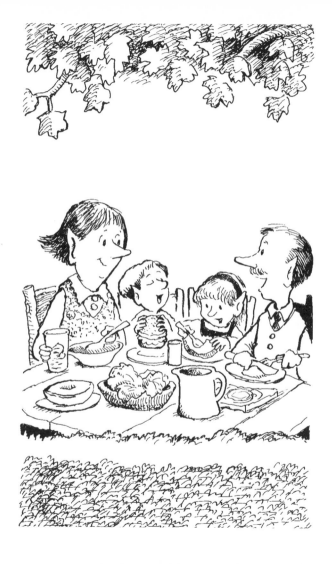

7.

Nourishment is not just what you put in your mouth. We create health daily not just by eating well but by maintaining balance in our work, exercise, relationships, play, rest, and spiritual practice.

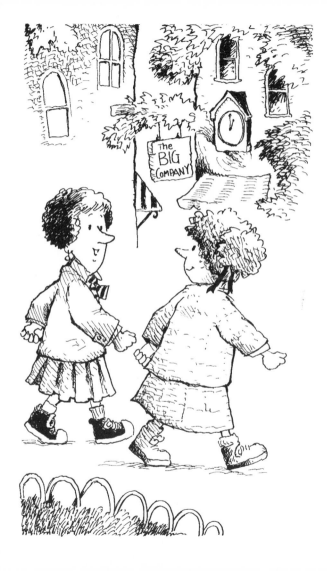

8.

When you cultivate love in your life through healthy relationships and spiritual practice, you create life-sustaining "primary food." This is the food of spirit that empowers you. The less of this "primary food" you have, the more you will rely on physical food for comfort, and the less happy you may be.

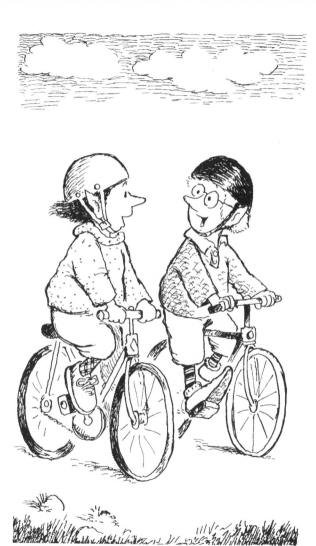

9.

In our fast-paced world, we can become desensitized to the earth and the food that is borne of it, and we forget to marvel at its life cycle. If you can, visit a farm where there are animals and crops. Appreciate the sun, water, and energy that go into cultivating the plants and animals that become our food.

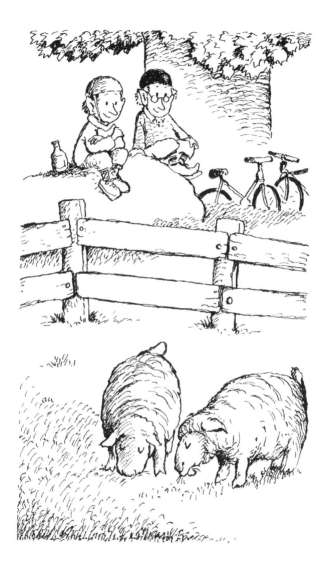

10.

Eat simple, natural foods that are close to the source. The simpler, less processed food we eat, the better for us. Eat foods that are grown seasonally and locally. Read labels—if a label has too many words you can't pronounce, you can be sure the item has been processed with additives that may be harmful.

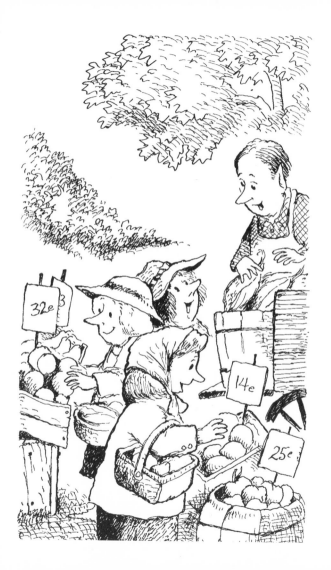

11.

While eating out may be easier and quicker, cooking at home means taking charge of your food preparation. You add love and awareness to the basic ingredients, and you create a beautiful masterpiece that nourishes and blesses all those who partake.

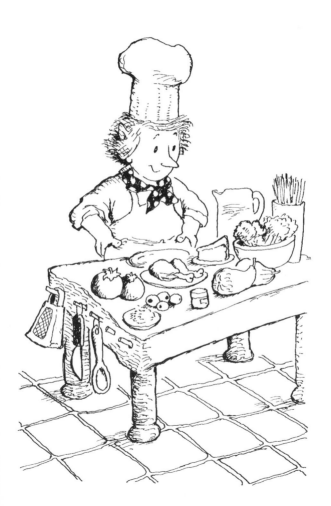

12.

Carefully moderate your intake of sugar, salt, and caffeine. It's not about the calories. These substances in excess can make us prone to debilitating conditions. (Be aware: sugar has many other names!) If you have recently quit one of these substances, be gentle and patient with yourself.

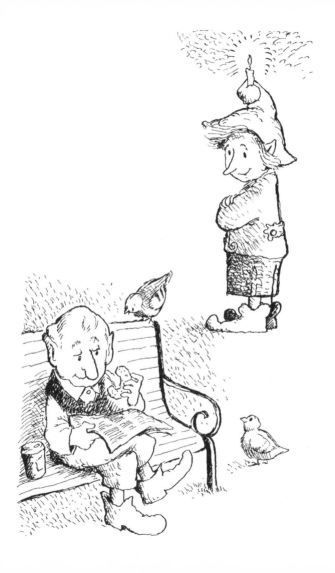

13.

Eat a lot of cooked, sweet vegetables like carrots, sweet potatoes, squash, beets, and onions when you are decreasing sugar intake. These foods help appease your sweet tooth and they actually help fight sugar cravings.

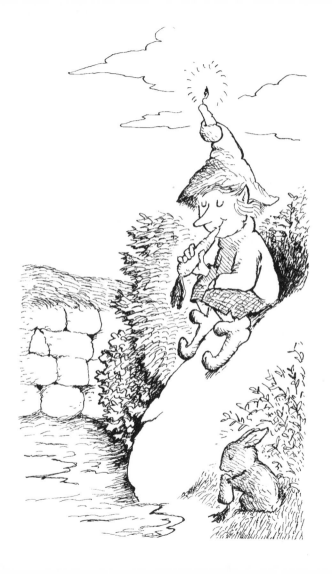

14.

Some of us are sensitive to dairy products without realizing it. We may develop symptoms like headaches, skin eruptions, and digestive disorders without realizing the connection. Calcium comes in other healthy alternatives such as greens (broccoli, kale, collards), beans, nuts, and seeds.

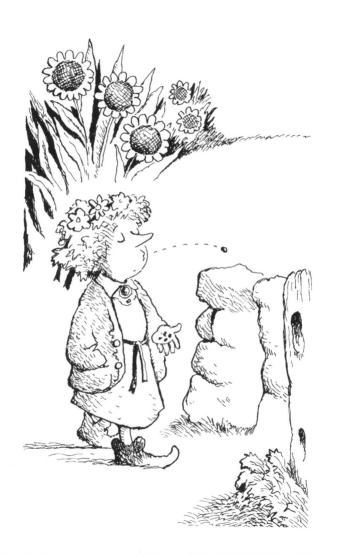

15.

Eat less animal foods and more fish, grains, legumes, vegetables, and fruit. These will provide a bounty of vitamins and nutrients.

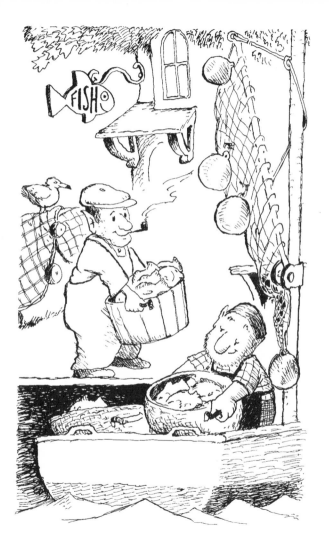

16.

Drink plenty of water. It is our life source! Sometimes when we're dehydrated we get irritable or we think we're hungry when all we need is a simple glass of water.

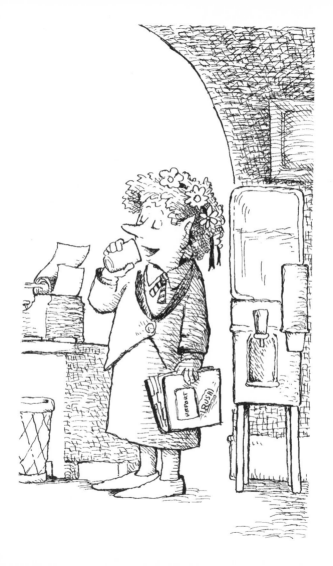

17.

Eat balanced amounts of protein, carbohydrates, and fats. Proteins are in fish and animal foods, but also in nuts and legumes. Fats have a bad reputation, but they are not all "bad"—olive oil, avocados, and nuts are actually relatively beneficial.

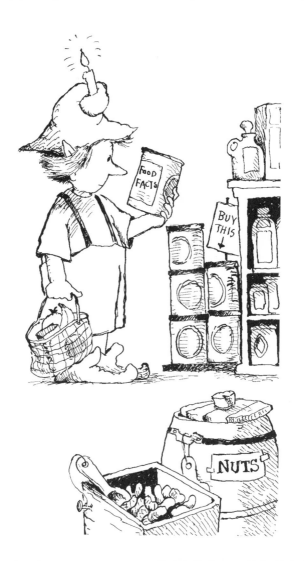

18.

Go on a beautiful "rainbow diet." Include at least four to five naturally occurring, colorful foods on the plate; the brighter the colors, the better (you'll get plenty of vitamins and fiber). Colorful foods include carrots, broccoli, yellow peppers, leafy greens, beets, sweet potatoes, beans, corn, and the list goes on!

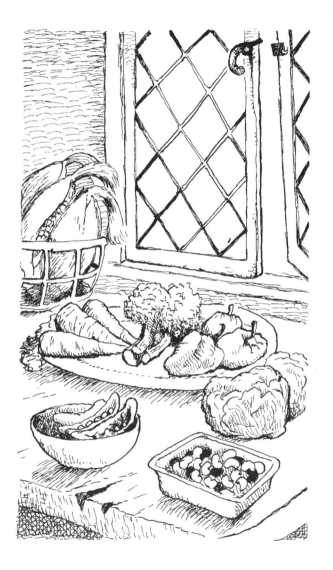

19.

Food can bring people together. Everybody eats, and cooking, sharing, and talking about foods from other cultures is a wonderful way to meet people and to appreciate other traditions.

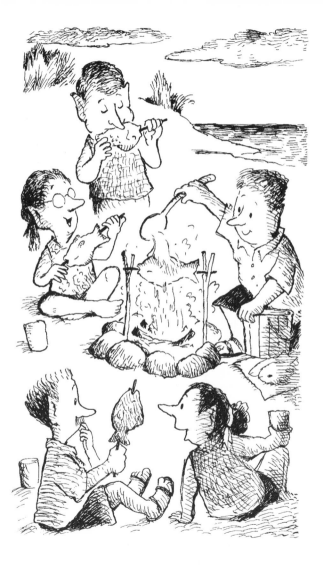

20.

Get your friends and family involved in the cooking process. Food and health are about community—a physical, spiritual, and emotional celebration.

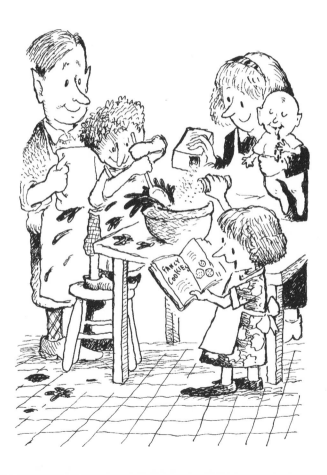

21.

Consider fasting—or at least eating less—for a day (no extremes). Don't think of it as a deprivation. Abstaining from consuming solid foods serves a spiritual and physical purpose. It is an opportunity for your body to recharge and reenergize. Remember to drink plenty of water and consult with a doctor beforehand.

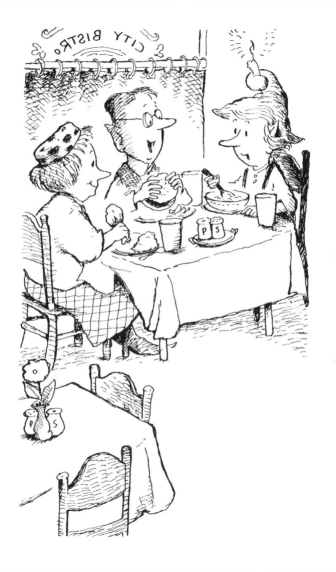

22.

Your body is a sanctuary. Treat it with reverence and love. As much as possible, eat the best quality foods available. Avoid processed, refined foods, and consider eating organic fruits, vegetables, and free-range animals that have not been subjected to pesticides, hormones, and antibiotics.

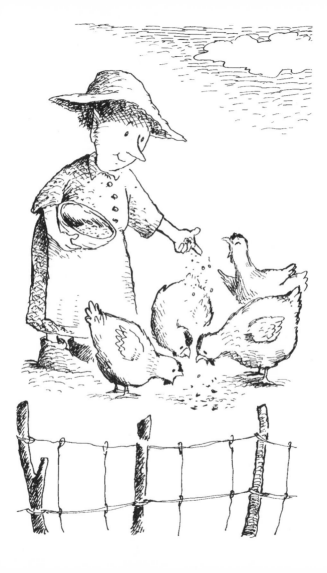

23.

Remember to practice good oral hygiene, which includes regular brushing and flossing. A clean mouth helps to remind you of your commitment to eating consciously.

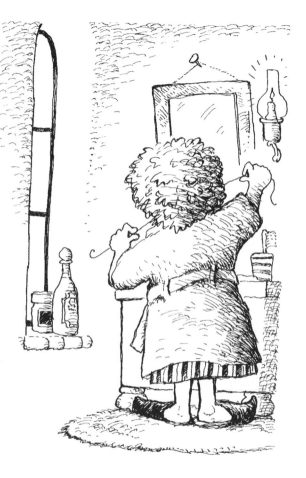

24.

When you eat, sit down at the table and look at your food with appreciation, and without distractions such as television, etc. Chew slowly and with awareness. You'll see that this simple ritual act will improve your digestion and provide you with greater clarity throughout the day.

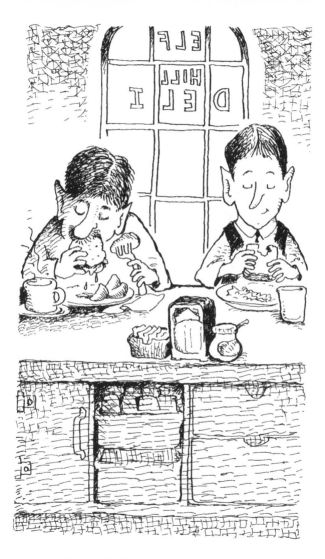

25.

When we eat out, we are at the mercy of other people's energy, food preparation, and portions. One way to regain power is to be aware of the ingredients and cooking process of the foods we eat, and to consume only what we feel comfortable eating.

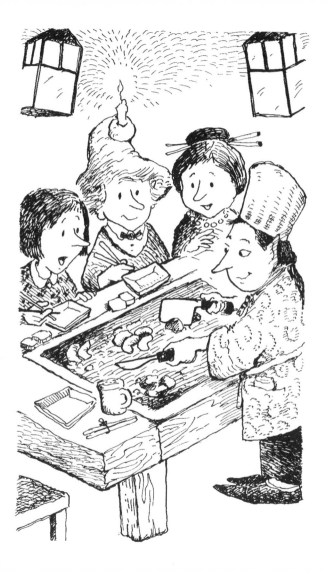

26.

Eat balanced meals at regular intervals during the day, and don't skip breakfast! Remember: fruits and vegetables make wonderful snacks.

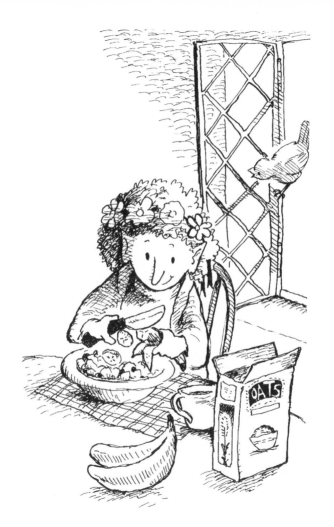

27.

Don't hide your emotions behind food. Emptiness, pain, numbness, and anger won't go away if we try to stuff these feelings down with food. Make a commitment to resolve past issues that drive you towards unhealthy, un-conscious eating.

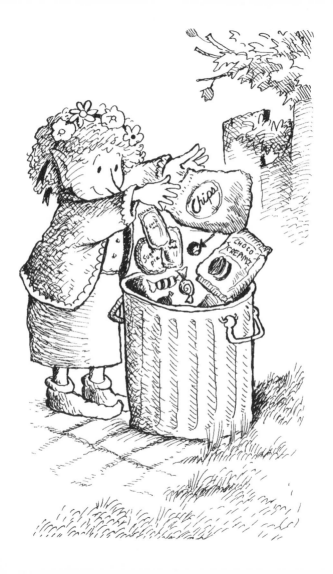

28.

Food is not a religion and nutrition is not about deprivation, reward, or punishment. All food is, by nature, "neutral." Food is simply a means to achieving and maintaining health so you can live to the fullest.

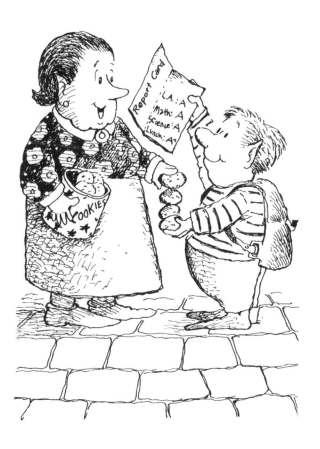

29.

Avoid thinking about food as "good" or "bad"—or yourself as "good" or "bad" when you eat specific foods. If you suspect you have become too rigid about food, or if you feel you may have an eating disorder, get help. Ask for the tools and information you need.

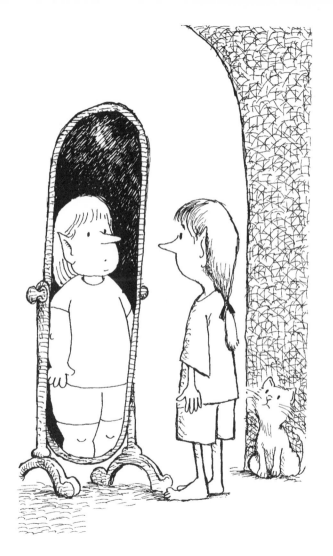

30.

If you make poor food choices on a particular day, don't beat yourself up about it. Try again the next day! Eating well isn't all or nothing. Dietary and lifestyle changes happen one small step at a time.

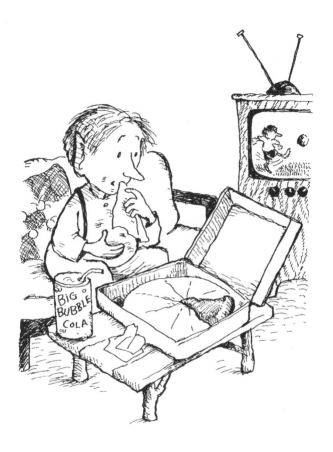

31.

Live in the present. Eat joyfully. Once in a while, if you feel like having a treat, indulge, but do so mindfully. Savor each bite and really enjoy the flavor. As soon as you are satisfied, stop.

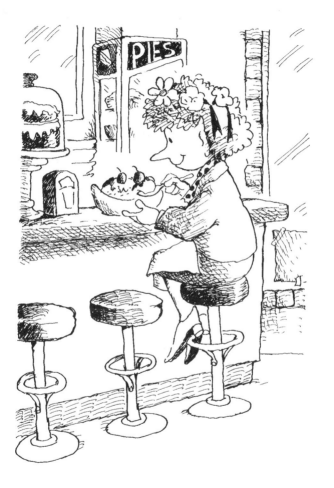

32.

Avoid eating mechanically, when you are sad, angry, bored, or tired. In these cases, instead of eating, you are "being eaten," and this symptom will show up on your body in one form or another.

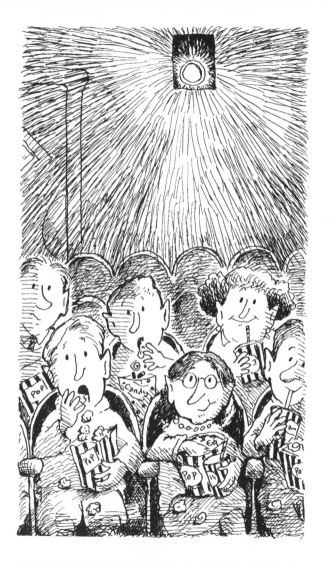

33.

Find nutrition buddies with whom you can share your commitment to eating more healthily. Share tips, ideas, recipes, and give each other support during life's ups and downs.

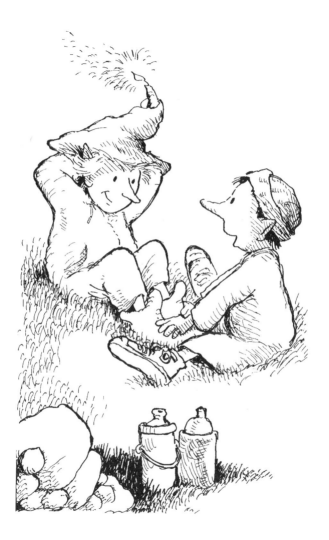

34.

Think positively—laugh,
engage your creativity,
do work you love, feed your
mind with good thoughts.
Play. Hug yourself and
others on a regular basis.

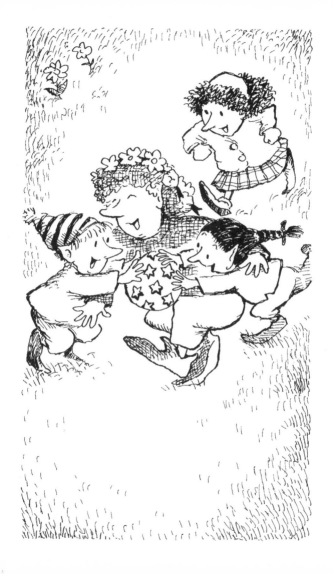

35.

Avoid negative people, gossip, and activities that "eat at you" and take away your energy and health. Similarly, be compassionate and caring with your own words and actions, and you'll "feed" the world with your wholesome goodness.

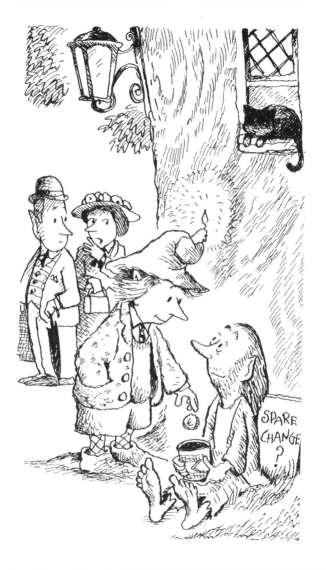

36.

Throughout the day, sing, pray out loud, laugh—feel the vibrations from your vocal cords all the way down to your belly. Joyful sounds stimulate and promote health to our digestive systems.

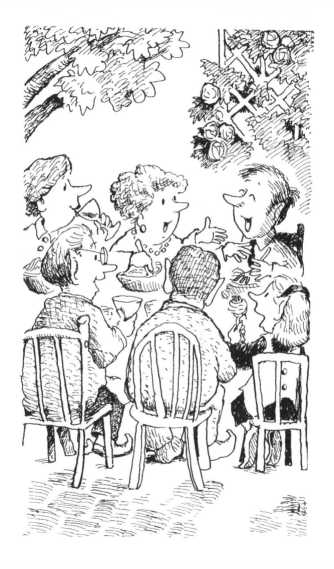

37.

Food and health are part of a process that is ever changing and never-ending. As we grow older, our bodies change and we develop different nutritional needs. Make a commitment to work continually towards achieving balance and well being through conscious eating.

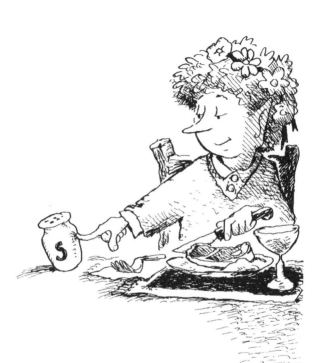

38.

Food is one of God's ways
of loving and nurturing us.
We make ourselves even more
mindful of this when we
give thanks!

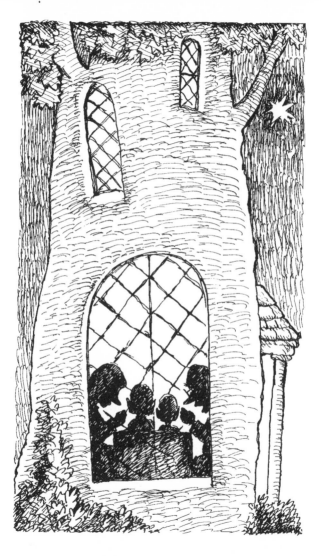

Laura E. Pirott received training in nutrition and holistic health counseling from the Institute for Integrative Nutrition in New York City. She is a professor of modern languages and currently teaches at the City University of New York. She loves to practice yoga, Tae Kwon Do, and to eat—of course!

Illustrator for the Abbey Press Elf-help Books, **R.W. Alley** also illustrates and writes children's books. He lives in Barrington, Rhode Island, with his wife, daughter, and son. See a wide variety of his works at: www.rwalley.com.

The Story of the Abbey Press Elves

The engaging figures that populate the Abbey Press "elf-help" line of publications and products first appeared in 1987 on the pages of a small self-help book called *Be-good-to-yourself Therapy*. Shaped by the publishing staff's vision and defined in R.W. Alley's inventive illustrations, they lived out the author's gentle, self-nurturing advice with charm, poignancy, and humor.

Reader response was so enthusiastic that more Elf-help Books were soon under way, a still-growing series that has inspired a line of related gift products.

The especially endearing character featured in the early books—sporting a cap with a mood-changing candle in its peak—has since been joined by a spirited female elf with flowers in her hair.

These two exuberant, sensitive, resourceful, kindhearted, lovable sprites, along with their lively elfin community, reveal what's truly important as they offer messages of joy and wonder, playfulness and co-creation, wholeness and serenity, the miracle of life and the mystery of God's love.

With wisdom and whimsy, these little creatures with long noses demonstrate the elf-help way to a rich and fulfilling life.

Elf-help Books

...adding "a little character" and a lot of help to self-help reading!

Friendship Therapy	#20174
Christmas Therapy (color edition) $5.95	#20175
Happy Birthday Therapy	#20181
Forgiveness Therapy	#20184
Keep-life-simple Therapy	#20185
Acceptance Therapy	#20190
Keeping-up-your-spirits Therapy	#20195
Slow-down Therapy	#20203
One-day-at-a-time Therapy	#20204
Prayer Therapy	#20206
Be-good-to-your-marriage Therapy	#20205
Be-good-to-yourself Therapy	#20255

Book price is $4.95 unless otherwise noted.
Available at your favorite gift shop or bookstore—
or directly from One Caring Place, Abbey Press
Publications, St. Meinrad, IN 47577.
Or call 1-800-325-2511.
www.carenotes.com